Reverse Diabetes

Lower Blood Sugar Levels Naturally and Live a Normal Life!

By

Dermot Farrell

www.healbodymindandspirit.com

MEDICAL DISCLAIMER

The information in this book is not intended to replace professional medical supervision. The information in this book is highly effective and it will definitely reduce and possible even reverse high blood sugar levels in most individuals. In some cases a cure may take place, however, there is no guarantee that physical ailments will be completely cured. Prior to reducing or stopping allopathic medications, do consult with a qualified physician.

Contents

PART TWO

REVERSING DIABETES

Foreword

Diabetes has reached epidemic levels with 9.3% of Americans over the age of 18 suffering with diabetes and according to the World health organization (WHO) 8.5% of the world population have with diabetes! These are ridiculous figures and clearly diabetes is out of control. But what can we do about it?

Diabetes is a complex health condition because diabetes can be split between type 1 which is genetically predetermined and it originates in childhood and appears to be unpreventable and type 2 diabetes, which appears during adulthood and is a mix of genetics and lifestyle. So in answer to the question what can we do about diabetes, there is no clear cut answer as some people develop diabetes against all odds largely, because of their genetics, however, for most of us we can either prevent diabetes from developing or at the very least we can reverse the symptomology of diabetes.

For a start if you are a prediabetic definitely diabetes can be prevented from developing, but what about if you have already developed diabetes, can it be reversed?

To be perfectly honest about it technically speaking apart from a miracle taking place, the biological damage which occurs in full blown diabetes cannot be reversed. Basically when a person develops full blown diabetes, the pancreas is not producing enough beta cells, which are required to produce insulin in the body. The medical specialists who work in diabetology, are working on ways to promote beta cell production or even the possibility of beta cell implant surgery, but as of yet once damaged they are largely unfixable. So what's all this talk about reversing diabetes then?

I wanted to address this in the foreword, as there are a lot of books about there which talk about reversing diabetes and sometimes it comes across that one can fix diabetes with a few lifestyle changes and that then the diabetes is completely cured!

But really if anyone could guarantee a scientifically provable cure, they would have the proof posted all over the internet and they would be regular visitors on premier TV shows!

In reality save for a miracle, a diabetic is still a diabetic even if they reverse the symptoms. So really when we speak about reversing diabetes, we are actually talking about reversing the symptoms of diabetes and living a symptom free happy and healthy life. This is quite possible, but technically speaking damage is still there and if the person who cures themselves, of the symptoms of diabetes starts eating a lot of simple carbohydrates and leading an inactive lifestyle, they will again develop the symptoms of diabetes!

I wanted to get this out into the open in the foreword of the book, as I feel it is reckless to set up an unrealistic expectation. Can you cure yourself of diabetes? Yes you can in the sense that you can be symptom free, but you have to be disciplined regarding food, supplements and exercise for the rest of your life, for some organic damage is still there if full blown diabetes has been initiated for more than a few months!

As noted earlier if you are a borderline diabetic, it can be completely reversed but if you have had full-blown diabetes for a few months or more, then you can be free of the symptoms but you have to be disciplined if you want to maintain your health and be symptom free going forward!

Is it worth your effort?

Certainly it's worth your while taking the time out to reverse the symptoms of diabetes. You might not convince an endocrinologist if he takes out detailed tests, but who cares! What matters with diabetes is protecting your health from long-term damage, by getting your sugar levels back under control and also freeing yourself of the discomfort of the symptoms of diabetes, which are infringing upon your life and will continue to become worse over time, unless you take charge now.

Diabetic medications, such as pills which are designed to help stimulate the beta cells and insulin for diabetics who have no beta cells, are all there to assist the diabetic patient, but really they are there just to prevent death from occurring as a consequence of sugar levels, which are either too low or too high. But ask any diabetic doctor and they will tell you that lifestyle changes have to be made, if you want to have a better quality of life and also in order to prevent further organic damage and negative side effects from taking place.

In reverse diabetes we are going to build upon this base as suggested by allopathic doctors, but we are also going to go one step further and look at super foods, herbal remedies, hatha yoga techniques, pranayama techniques and Taoist yoga techniques and even acupressure techniques, which will all go one step beyond the basic advice and if you stick with these techniques, while watching your diet, yes you can reverse the symptoms of diabetes, which will empower you to lead a normal healthy life, which is free of diabetic symptoms and which will be largely protected from the long-term degenerative effects of diabetes!

Part One – Understanding Diabetes

Chapter One – Understanding Diabetes Type 1 and Type 2

Diabetes is on the rise throughout the world and according to the World Health organization (WHO) it is the sixth largest cause of death in the world reporting a total of 1.3 million deaths in 2015 coming about as a result of diabetes!

Diabetes can start out as a relatively minor health condition, but over time it can result in a lot of degenerative health conditions. The most obviously acute health condition is ketogenic coma which comes about as a consequence of sugar levels which are too low to maintain brain health (two thirds of our bodies glucose goes to feed our Bain which runs on glycogen). But there are other less obvious health conditions which come about as a consequence of diabetes, which are:

- Fungal infections

- Skin problems

- Urinary tract infections

- High blood pressure

- Heart disease

- Kidney disease

- Retinopathy (damage to the retina in the eyes)

- Neuropathy (damage to the nerves in the skin)

- Ketogenic coma

- Blood clots resulting in amputation/sudden death

At a simple level when a person becomes diabetic, they have difficulty dealing with sugar. Sugar is found everywhere, not just in table sugar but rather in all carbohydrates. Carbohydrates are a major food macronutrient (the other two been protein and fat). Carbohydrates can then be split into simple (fast acting) and complex (slow acting). Our bodies use carbohydrates for fuel, but in the case of diabetics, either the body does not produce enough insulin or the insulin is ineffective at processing the sugar into a form which can be absorbed by our cells. As a consequence of this we can either suffer with too little sugar or too much sugar in our blood.

Too little sugar and we can go into a coma and too much sugar will ravage our cardiovascular system which in turn can result in damage to the kidneys and other organs where blood supply is required, such as the eyes and the skin.

While most people can control their sugar levels with relative ease via pills or insulin, over time the sugar levels tend to be reside above normal which result in a higher HB1Ac reading. This is a reading of our baseline blood sugar levels, taken over a period of months. This is a little different from the blood glucose reading, which we can take on a regular basis via a blood testing kit. Normally a diabetic's blood sugar levels are a little high, but by regular monitoring via a blood sugar testing unit they can adjust their drug intake so as to normalise their daily blood levels. But even though they may manage to maintain ok(ish) blood sugar levels most of the time, much of the time blood sugar levels will still be elevated, although the diabetic patient will get used to this and accept the feelings of fatigue and frequent fungal infections and skin itching sensations which go with this as normal, but nonetheless damage is been carried out and when we take the HB1Ac reading we can easily see an elevated sugar level over a period of months. What this means is that slowly over a period of months and year's damage is taken place to the cardiovascular system which in turn will lead onto the degenerative conditions mentioned above.

Common side effects of diabetes includes skin rashes (usually caused by fungal infections as a consequence of high blood sugar levels), itching in the skin and fatigue. Other longer term side effects include a variety of skin problems and also the potential for such conditions as damage to the vision and neuropathy, which can result in numbness in the feet, for example, also neuropathy result in severe pins and needles sensation in the feet, which can be very painful. Numbness in the feet often results in the feet getting cut without the diabetic patient realising this, which can turn dangerous over time, especially since the cardiovascular damage makes recovery of the damaged part of the foot impossible. Often if not taken care of this can result in amputation, which is a common occurrence in long term diabetic patients. Also amputation often promotes blood clots which can easily obstruct either the heart or the brain causing death!

Also heart damage, leading onto heart attacks and kidney damage resulting in kidney organ failure can also result!

So we cannot underestimate the devastating effects of diabetes vote the long-term!

But there is light at the end of the tunnel, in that even if you have been suffering from diabetes for many years, you can take charge of the situation and reverse it thus preventing further damage from taken place. Now if damage has already occurred you cannot turn back time and undo it, but you can take things in hand and prevent further damage from occurring. Going back it the HB1Ac by following the instructions in this book and been strict about it, you can regularise your fasting sugar levels and this doesn't just mean your daily sugar levels rather it also means your sugar levels over a period of months. Once sugar levels have properly stabilised over a period of time the damage will stop!

Furthermore the supplements and herbs mentioned can go a long way to protecting your body against many of the nasty long-term side effects associated with diabetes!

The single most important step lies in getting your sugar levels under control and alleviation of symptoms will follow on from this. But first let's take a quick look at the types and causes of diabetes.

Type 1 Diabetes

Type 1 diabetes kicks off in childhood and is an autoimmune disease whereby the immune system kills of the beta cells in the pancreas, which in turn makes it impossible to properly process sugars in the body.

The causes of type 1 diabetes are not clear. It is suggested that the probably causes are:

- Viral or bacterial infection

- Chemical toxins in the foods which we eat

- Genetic predisposition

While it is unclear why exactly some children develop this condition, the most noticeable difference between type 1 diabetes and type 2 diabetes is that with type 2 diabetes, lifestyle appears to have a very significant effect on the aetiology of the condition, whereas with type one diabetes, it appears to strike suddenly even in the most active and slim kids, who have a good diet and an active lifestyle!

Type 2 Diabetes

Type 2 diabetes also has a genetic component but lifestyle appears to be a much stronger determinant factor. The likely causes of type2 diabetes are:

- Obesity

- Sedentary Living

- Age

- Genetics

Type 1 diabetes then can be seen as an unfortunate incident whereas by and large type 2 diabetes reflects a lifestyle which is low on activity and high on simple carbohydrates, which when combined with a genetic predisposition will result in diabetes.

There are of course some individuals who are very inactive, obese and who eat a terribly diet and yet they will never suffer from diabetes, but that is the luck of the genetic draw as it were. In general a sedentary lifestyle which is based upon an abundance of fast acting carbohydrates and highly processed foods, is a recipe for disaster which will invariably result in either the onset of diabetes, heart disease or both diabetes and heart disease.

Differences Between Type 1 and Type 2 Diabetes?

By and large bath type 1 and type 2 diabetes are similar in action in that the body is unable to effectively process sugar in the body but there are a few differences:

1. In type 1 diabetes the beta cells are completely destroyed resulting in the necessity of taking insulin injections. Usually with type 2 diabetes, diabetic medications can stimulate the beta cells to some degree, although some type 2 diabetic have to take insulin. The insulin which is supplied to diabetics is an exact copy of the insulin in the human body, although depending upon how it is processed the delivery time's f this insulin may vary. The biggest challenge with insulin is that if the diabetic patient takes too much they can end up in a coma, if they are not careful!

2. Type 1 diabetes usually occurs during childhood or young adulthood, whereas type 2 diabetes occurs later in life. In the past many people developed type 2 diabetes in their sixties but today, thanks to an unhealthy lifestyle many people are developing type 2 diabetes in the thirties and even in their twenties. If you are a young person or know a young person with a sedentary lifestyle and a very junkie diet, then there is a good chance that they will develop diabetes if they're not careful.

3. With type 1 diabetes it is very common to have episodes of low blood sugar because the insulin when is injected, if a little too much is taken, will result in hypoglycaemia. This occurs because exogenous (externally

received) insulin delivery is not exact and it impedes the glucose counter regularity system, thus bringing about hypoglycaemia, which can result in the onset of coma in some cases. This can also take place sometimes in type 2 diabetes, but it is a far less frequent occurrence, as the glucose counter regularity system is usually intact in type 2 diabetics. This mechanism is an automatic regulatory system in the human body which is designed to stop the body going into hypoglycaemia. In hypoglycaemia the bodies sugar levels fall drastically, resulting in a lack of glucose reaching the brain which in turn promotes the onset of a coma and can in same cases result in death. Normally when the sugar levels drop, the body releases sugars from the liver into the bloodstream in order to promote a stable blood sugar level, but this is very often lacking in type 1 diabetics.

4. As of yet type 1 diabetes cannot be prevented, whereas type 2 diabetes is largely created as a consequence of diet and lifestyle. In fairness many diabetics would become diabetics sooner or later, thanks to their genetics but there is a big difference in becoming a diabetic at seventy years of age and becoming a diabetic at twenty seven!

5. Type 1 diabetics usually suffer with more severe health problems as a consequence of their diabetes, starting at an earlier age and also because of the complete lack of insulin, often it is a more severe type of diabetes in the first place. As a rule of thumb the longer one is a diabetic, the worse the side effects. So a person who develops diabetes at age sixty will probably only have to take one pill a day and often will have very few side effects, whereas a person who becomes a diabetic at age ten might well have extensive degenerative problems by the time they reach sixty, if they reach sixty, which could include organ failure and possible amputations!

In summary just about anyone can potentially become a diabetic patient, if their lifestyle is extremely unhealthy, although in most cases there is a strong genetic determinant.

This leads onto the obvious question, can diabetes be avoided?

Clearly in type 1 diabetes it cannot be avoided. Maybe at some stage a clear cause will be pinpointed and maybe then it can be prevented, but for now there is nothing which can be done. Regarding type 2 diabetes, in many cases it can be completely avoided and even where it cannot be avoided, it can be put of to a late stage in life. A very important consideration in diabetes is that the longer on has it the greater the level of organic damage. So while some peoples genetic predestination towards diabetes is very strong, it can certainly be put off to a very later age.

Also there is the subject of:

Prediabetes

Prediabetes is extremely common these days and if you are prediabetic or know anyone who is then cheer up or cheer them up because at this stage full blown diabetes is very avoidable. In the prediabetic stages the body is just starting to lose control as the body struggles with insulin resistance, whereby either there is not enough insulin or the insulin doesn't work effectively at getting the cells to absorb the sugars. Insulin resistance is a common occurrence on account of a diet which is very high in simple sugars. As a result of this diet the body has to keep spewing out large doses of insulin, which can wear out the pancreas beta cells over time, or in many cases the cells of the body simply become resistant to the vast amount of insulin in the blood stream and as such the person starts to develop diabetic symptoms.

Atypically the prediabetic blood sugar levels are in the borderline range, whereby fasting sugar levels are a little on the high side.

The good news is that reducing simple carbohydrate intake and increasing exercise, will often do the trick. Something as simple as going to the gym every day or performing a sporting activity such as tennis or badminton or an athletic activity such as swimming, will often do the trick. If your health or time is lacking you could of course go for a gentle walk, but really to get the best stimulation you should perform some fairly intense exercise.

Also another good tactic for the prediabetic, is the use some intermittent fasting so as to stimulate human growth hormone levels in the body. When you go a good few hours without food (around twelve to sixteen depending upon the person) the human growth hormone (HGH) levels will peak and when they peak insulin levels have to be low. Now I know you might be thinking that as a prediabetic you need more insulin and not less but the whole problem with prediabetics is that their bodies are usually insulin resistant. By taking a couple of days in a week and doing some light (twelve to sixteen hours) of intermittent fasting, often this will reset the body within a few weeks, so that when combined with exercise the insulin resistance will go away!

Now this tactic won't work on full blown diabetics, who have to eat every few hours simply to maintain blood sugar levels, but it does work great on rape prediabetics!

So onto the next big question can we reverse diabetes and if so how?

Chapter Two – How Can We Reverse Diabetes?

As noted in the foreword, the whole concept of reverse diabetes is a bit of misnomer. Basically if anyone could scientifically demonstrate a complete reversal of diabetes, they would obviously be posting the results everywhere from the TV to the internet!

So obviously no one can fully reverse diabetes, to the degree that there are absolutely no signs of diabetes (as in the beta cells have recovered), because to do so would be a miracle. Rather what can take place is that the symptoms can be completely reversed (if you start the recovery process in the early stages of diabetes), to the degree that even the HB1Ac results are in the normal range. The beta cells will still be damaged, although in some cases some degree of recovery might take place, but not back to normal levels, unless a miracle does take place (which happens every now and again!).

So there are two groups on opposing sides of the fence. On one side we have the medical authorities who strongly suggest lifestyle changes but who totally disbelieve that diabetes can be reversed in any shape or form, and on the other side we have ardent complementary therapists who believe that of course diabetes is completely curably, as really it's not a disease rather it's a simple imbalance!

I'm not knocking complementary therapists, after all I am one myself, but let's face it in any case of full blown diabetes (not prediabetes) the beta cells have become permanently damaged and short of a miracle they're never going to return back to normal! So it's one thing which irks me about complementary healthcare, is the tendency to throw everything into a convenient but vague and inaccurate label. Sure most diabetics have become diabetic because of poor lifestyle choices, but many people would end up there anyhow due to genetic predisposition, maybe not now but at some stage in the future!

Also I don't favour the medical authorities and their pessimism either, whereby they hand out nice little pamphlets labelled with unhelpful suggestions such as "living with Diabetes" as if that's it you're stuck with it now for life.

So if you have just been labelled a diabetic, there is a slim chance that you may be able to completely reverse your diabetes and make a complete cure. If you have been diabetic for a while and are definitely beyond the prediabetic stages, then you can become free of the symptoms, but technically speaking there is objective damage to the cells in the pancreas, which mean that the only way in which you can maintain you health is through a strict diet and an active lifestyle. Whereas prediabetics might get away with the odd big splurge of junk food, without any fear of after effects, for the recovering full blown diabetic junk food outings will take at least several days for the blood sugars to return back to normal, and of course if you eat a lot of junk you will find yourself back into the land of uncontrolled sugar levels once more!

What about Type 1 Diabetics and Long-Term Diabetic Patients?

Definitely if you are type 1 diabetic or a long term diabetic patient, it is worth your while following the steps outlined in this book, perhaps even more so that the prediabetic or the fairly new diabetic patient, for with long-term diabetes comes many degenerative side effects, which really need to be addressed!

While it may not be completely possible to reverse all symptoms of diabetes, there is an urgent need for long-term type 2 and type 1 diabetics to get their diabetes under control, so as to prevent the acute side effects of diabetes such as organ failure, amputations, clots etc.!

So in an ideal world we can all hope for a complete and perfect recovery, but obviously when dealing with a health condition which effects 8% of the world's adult population, there is going to be a wide degree of variance between different people, but certainly full reversal is possible in some cases and in all cases a great improvement can be made!

Is Diabetes a Disease?

This is a moot question for the allopathic medical fraternity likes to stick to their labels, whereas complementary therapists and complementary dieticians will see diabetes as a health condition or syndrome. In a way both groups are right, in that from the perspective of dead beta cells, in the pancreas, certainly diabetes is a disease and from the perspective of a syndrome, much of what we call prediabetic behaviour is the body struggling to deal with a vast influx of simple carbohydrates and lack of exercise!

Both perspectives have their merits. For a start let's get real, if your beta cells are damaged the days of pigging out and getting away with it are over, you simply have to be strict with your diet, if you want to maintain your blood sugar levels in the normal range for both fasting sugars and Hb1Ac also. Also from the syndrome point of view the good thing to take away from this, is to stop labelling yourself, yes you might have insulin resistance and damaged beta cells, but does this define you as a human being? Of course not you can turn things around, long-term degeneration is not inevitable!

So How Do we go About Reversing Diabetes?

The process of reversal begins with following the standard advice given by your doctor and then take everything a stage or two further. Your doctor will suggest a healthy diet and exercise. Well we're simply going to recommend the same while making some specific notes about diet which doctor might not have outlined in detail and we will be looking in detail both at super foods and herbal supplements, which will greatly help to balance not only sugar levels but also they can be a great help in protecting the body against the onset of many of the degenerative illnesses which come along with diabetes!

Also from the exercise point of view we shall take a look at some Hatha yoga techniques, Taoist yoga techniques and Pranayama breathing as well as regular exercises. Also we shall take a look at some acupressure points, which will assist you on your journey towards normalising baseline sugar levels and reversing the symptoms of diabetes!

In part two a chapter shall be laid out on each of these areas noted above and a final concluding chapter shall provide you with some solid advice as to the best way to roll out this diabetes reversal plan!

Coming of Diabetic Medications?

This is a very important consideration, for if you are to reverse your diabetes, a stage must come in most cases where diabetic medications are reduced. However, this is going to vary a lot from person to person. A person with type 1 diabetes is basically going to have to take exogenous insulin whether they like it or not as they have no working beta cells left. So in their case they are looking at improving HB1Ac levels to the point that baseline sugar levels are normalised, even over the long term. Once again to reiterate the difference between fasting blood sugar levels and HB1Ac levels, fasting blood sugar only refers to blood sugar levels first thing in the morning on an empty stomach whereas Hb1Ac refers to blood sugars as a baseline, which is a far deeper thing. You may well have normalish blood sugar levels in the morning but then once you eat they rise substantially. However, when the HB1Ac result comes back within the normal range it means that blood sugars are well controlled all of the time!

28

So for someone with very serious degeneration in the beta cells, the aim is to become symptom free, so take as much insulin as is required. For the problem which most type 1 diabetics and long-term type 2 diabetics is that they tend to have to take a lot of insulin, but their HB1Ac is all over the place and even their daily fasting sugars are really bad. So in this case taking insulin is a must, but first of all getting the daily fasting sugars right and then moving onto normalising the HB1Ac levels over time.

For type 2 diabetics and prediabetics, it is a different ball gaming altogether. In the case of prediabetics they are not taking pills anyway and in the case of most type 2 diabetics, they are usually taking one pill a day and in some cases insulin is also required. The mature approach towards reducing drug intake, is to start with daily monitoring of blood sugar levels. You must monitor your levels and as the fasting levels start to reflect a normal range then start reducing pills, by reducing to maybe three quarter of a pill a day and so on over a period of days and weeks, dropping around quarter of a pill every few days and then monitoring daily to see how you are getting on. If everything keeps going down, then good and if instead fasting sugar levels start going back up again then increase the pill intake.

An example of pill reduction on one pills day

Week One – After seen several days in a row with normal fasting sugar levels drop down to three quarters of a pill. Simply break the pill into two and then the two pieces again into two and take three pieces instead of four.

Week Two – Fasting sugar levels still look good so now reduce down to half a pill per day.

Week Three – Fasting sugar levels still looking good so now reduce down to quarter of a pill per day.

Week Four – Fasting levels still looking good so reduce to zero pills per day.

The only way to gauge this is through trial and error, so keep on checking fasting sugar levels and see how you are doing. Fasting sugar levels are really important because most diabetics will take a pill once a day, so chances are that if you have taken a pill, say after your lynch, then by 7am the next morning that the pill has probably more or less left your system and now your actual baseline sugar levels are revealing themselves. Just remember to always go by fasting sugar levels, as sugar levels rafter meals will always be misleading. Also if you had a very heavy meal the night before, levels might be elevated slightly so bear that in mind too.

The best approach is to take out a notebook and maintain a daily record of your fasting sugar levels and for this you will need a glucose testing kit like the one in the picture below. Now from experience I can tell you that the single greatest mistake which I have seen diabetics make, over the years, is in not checking their sugar levels on a regular basis.

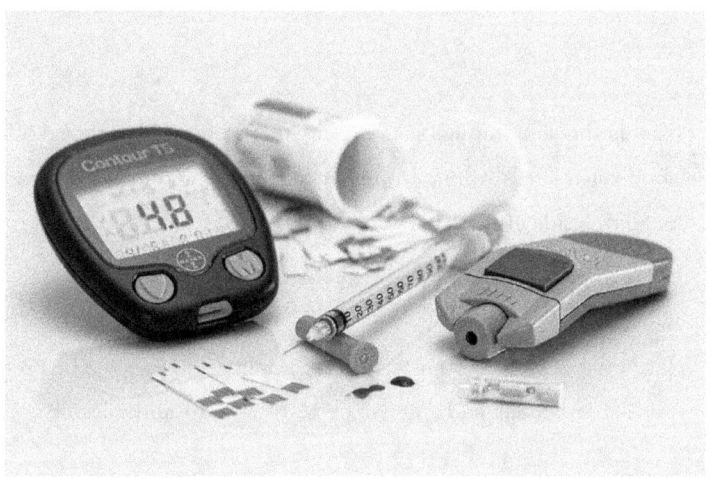

A Note on Checking Sugar Levels on a Regular Basis

How often should a diabetic check their sugar levels?

This will vary from person to person, but typically when a person first develops diabetes they should check on a daily basis and once they start getting things under control with medication they can reduce this down to a couple of times week. Also in some cases where diabetes is totally uncontrolled, it may be necessary to check blood sugar levels several times a day, although this is rare. Usually this is a rare case, but also it is common for people when they first go onto insulin to have to check several times a day, while they adjust their insulin intake.

What is shocking though is the reality that so many diabetics don't check their blood sugar levels from one season to the next and then they wonder why they are getting side effects!

Here's the deal, keep your fasting sugar inline and you will be pretty health, keep your HB1Ac inline and you will be 100% healthy and normal!

The way to do this for any diet, is by checking fasting blood sugar levels and taking it from there. Once your fasting sugar levels are good, every time you check then take an HB1Ac test. Perform it a couple of times a year, as it will show you how your blood sugar levels are normalising over a three month period. If you have a chance take an HB1Ac now and then takes one three months later and see if it has improved, as this is the real proof of improvement!

The goal of this book is reversal of diabetes and of course for prediabetis and people who have fairly early stage diabetic symptoms a complete reversal is often possible, but the only way to judge this is via the fasting blood sugar test taken regularly. Don't go by feel!

As a rule of thumb people feel really bad when their blood sugar levels go way out of control, but once they have been out of control for a while, most people won't feel bad at all unless they have strong symptoms, such as excessive fatigue, skin infections, and urinary tract infections and so on. The important thing here is that often a diabetic won't have many side effects for years, by which stage a lot of damage has already been done!

Also regarding early stage and later stage diabetics, this does not refer to how many years you have had diabetes, rather it refers to the severity of it. As a general rule of thumb, people who have had diabetes for a long time tend to have a lot of symptoms but then again there are people who have had diabetes for twenty years, but their debates is still very mild.

How then can we tell the difference?

The answer to this is simply how far out of synch are your blood sugar levels. If you have had diabetes for twenty years, but only take one pill a day and your fasting sugar levels are only elevated by say 20%, then chances are that you have early stage diabetes, whereas you could have diabetes for a year and yet your fasting sugars are five hundred present over normal and you have a plethora of symptoms and a team of doctors looking over your case, well in this case you have advanced stage diabetes!

Ok so what are normal fasting sugar levels and also what levels should we have after eating food?

Fasting Blood Sugar Levels		
Levels	Fasting	Two Hours After Eating (Postprandial)
Normal	100 mg/ld. (5.6 mol/L)	Under 140 mg/dl (7.8mmol/L)
Prediabetic	100 to 125 mg/dL (5.6 to 6.9 mmol/L)	Between 140 and 200mg/dL (7.8 and 11.1mmol/L)
Diabetic	126 mg/dL (7 mmol/L) or higher on two separate tests	Equal or above 200mg/dL (11.1mmol/L)

Of these are the daily fasting blood sugar levels but what about the HB1Ac?

HB1Ac Levels	
Levels	Fasting
Normal	4% and 5.6%
Prediabetic	5.7% and 6.4%
Diabetic	6.5% or higher

Interestingly when I Googled HB1Ac, in an effort to make up this table, the information which I came across states that once you are 6.5% or higher that you are diabetic and this is the sort of labelling of health conditions which we have to get away from. For if a diabetic patient manages to get into the lower range does this mean that they are not a diabetic?

So this is the problem with labelling diabetes, I am a firm believer that nearly all diabetics can get into the normal range of 4.6% to 5.6% on this test, although to do so will take discipline and consistency and some months so as to bring the blood sugars inline, but it's worth it because health benefits will comes about as a consequence of this!

So again to briefly summarise, for some diabetics insulin will be needed, so technically speaking they may never be cured of their diabetes, but they can get both their fasting sugars and HB1Ac in line, which means that they are normal. Whereas for others they can drop all medication and still come out fine on both of these tests. Whereas for some other people no matter how hard they try, their levels will still be somewhat elevated, but even so, they will greatly be able to reduce their fasting and HB1Ac levels which will go a long way towards reducing symptoms and protecting the body from long-term organic damage!

Finally even if you manage to completely reverse your diabetes don't throw out your diabetic testing kit, even if you check one or twice a month, it will be a good idea as once you have been prediabetic or mildly diabetic, your body will have a

35

tendency to go back towards diabetes. For the prediabetics once normalised, they can have pig out days and so on whereas for full-blown diabetics, who make a recovery, some organic damage will be there and a disciplined eye will have to be maintained on both diet and physical activity levels!

Part Two

Reversing Diabetes

Chapter Three – General Diet & Exercise Advice

Before taking a look at the more exotic approaches towards dealing with diabetes, let's take a brief look at the standard advice which your doctor will give you and take this as a starting point.

Let's take a quick look at recommendations which are made regarding the diet of diabetics by the According to the American Diabetes Association.

- If obese attempt to lose weight, as even a modest weight loss has a beneficial effect upon blood sugar levels. Although the effects of bodily fat levels on blood sugar levels is not clear, one thing is certain, that obese people tend to have more resistance to insulin than non-obese people, meaning that they need to have more insulin in their system to do the same amount of work.

- It is recommended to eat a diet which is rich in healthy fibre rich foods such as fruits, vegetables, legumes and whole grains, as fibre slows down the absorption of simple carbohydrates in the body. The problem with most processed foods these days is that they are high in simple carbohydrates, which in turn results in a sugar spikes, so eating lots of green leafy vegetables and healthy foods such as oats, for example, will help to reduce sugar spikes.

- It can be helpful to take a look at the glycemic index, as this reveals how quickly foods will release their sugar. Some foods, such as candy for example, are obviously high in quick releasing sugars, but do you know that say noodles, for example, are also high in quick releasing carbohydrates! This is an area where every diabetic patient has to get their head around their own bodies and the lifestyle choices which they make. A good starting place is taking a look at the foods you eat and seeing how they stack up according to the glycemic index (GI) chart. But also each person will have a slightly different result, out of eating the same foods, because of slight differences in the length and health of the small intestines, stomach health and efficiency levels and general blood chemistry. So start observing what you're eating and see how it affects you blood sugars after wards and adjust your diet accordingly.

Regarding Low-Carb and Low-Fat Diets

- It has been observed that diets which restrict carbohydrates or fat intake can reduce weight in the short-term (one year).
- The American Diabetes Association (ADA) has also noted that both low-carb and low-fat diets can work well and that the best approach is to use the diet which works for you, in other words the diet which you can stick to.
- Patients with kidney problems should limit their protein intake and should not substitute protein with carbohydrates, although patients who are on dialysis should take in more protein.

Glycemic Index

Low GI (<55), Medium GI (56-69) and High GI (70>)

Grains / Starchs		Vegetables		Fruits		Dairy		Proteins	
Rice Bran	27	Asparagus	15	Grapefruit	25	Low-Fat Yogurt	14	Peanuts	21
Bran Cereal	42	Broccoli	15	Apple	38	Plain Yogurt	14	Beans, Dried	40
Spaghetti	42	Celery	15	Peach	42	Whole Milk	27	Lentils	41
Corn, sweet	54	Cucumber	15	Orange	44	Soy Milk	30	Kidney Beans	41
Wild Rice	57	Lettuce	15	Grape	46	Fat-Free Milk	32	Split Peas	45
Sweet Potatoes	61	Peppers	15	Banana	54	Skim Milk	32	Lima Beans	46
White Rice	64	Spinach	15	Mango	56	Chocolate Milk	35	Chickpeas	47
Cous Cous	65	Tomatoes	15	Pineapple	66	Fruit Yogurt	36	Pinto Beans	55
Whole Wheat Bread	71	Chickpeas	33	Watermelon	72	Ice Cream	61	Black-Eyed Beans	59
Muesli	80	Cooked Carrots	39						
Baked Potatoes	85								
Oatmeal	87								
Taco Shells	97								
White Bread	100								
Bagel, White	103								

Ok say some generally good solid advice. But what can we add to this?

Macronutrients and Fat Intake and Nutritional Supplements for Diabetics

There are three main food groups which are labeled as macronutrients and these are proteins, carbohydrates and fats. Protein is required for building lean muscle mass, so all of our muscles, tissues and organs are reliant upon protein intake. Meanwhile both carbohydrates and fats are fuel for the body. The difference between carbohydrates and fats is that carbohydrates, especially simple carbohydrates raise blood sugar levels rapidly, whereas fats don't really raise blood sugar levels much unless you eat huge amounts of fats at one sitting.

Let's look at protein first. Protein is really important for maintaining muscle mass and for diabetics protein has to be taken seriously. For a start insulin deprivation has a catabolic effect on muscle mass, meaning that when a diabetic's natural insulin levels drops, muscle wasting starts to kick in. This can be a problem because over a period of time, as muscle levels drop it slows down the speed of the metabolism which in turn promotes obesity and can kick of diabetic symptoms. So there are two things which diabetics can do to help to prevent this or lessen this, and that is to exercise, ideally using resistance training (weight training) and also to maintain a decent protein intake.

So it is vital for diabetics to maintain good protein intake levels. However on the other side some diabetics have kidney damage, in which case protein levels should be rescued as it will worsen the health of the kidneys.

What about protein intake timings?

There is a common misconception that if you take your carbohydrates along with your protein that this will reduce the sugar spike, but evidence for this is lacking. The most up to date research suggests that protein spikes insulin and that the only advantage of combining carb intake with protein intake is that protein takes a longer time to be absorbed, so postprandial levels tend to demonstrate lower blood sugar levels, several hours after eating carbohydrates than eating carbs on their own. So really the only major reason for combining carbs and protein is to have balanced diet.

Also another consideration regarding protein is to not eat too much protein. For example a 100gram meal whether it is carbs, protein or carbs and proteins will result in a big blood sugar spike and will require quite a bit of insulin to process it. Now protein requires insulin to be absorbed, plus if you take a lot of protein the extra protein via the process of glycogenesis gets converted into carbohydrates!

So what can we take from this?

Basically make sure you're eating enough protein for health but not too much and do bear in mind that large amount of protein and carbs will spike sugar levels, so the best approach is to eat frequent small meals, so that the blood sugar spikes are smaller. Whenever you eat, there will be a sugar spike but we're looking for a smaller spike, so as to balance out sugar levels over time.

Regarding carb types, there are simple and complex, so ideally eat more complex than simple, which is pretty straight forward as in eat more unprocessed whole foods and less processed junkie types of foods, which is simple common sense. Also keep a watch on fruits, for while fruits are healthy and they are high in fructose, which is a healthier sugar than sucrose, they are still high in sugar and some people take loads of fruit, without releasing that their carbohydrate intakes are still very high and this will of course spike sugar levels over time.

Vegetables are really underestimated in that dark green leafy vegetables are high in fiber and although they possess carbs, the carbs which they possess are very slow releasing. So combining a lot of dark green leafy vegetables (salad and boiled or steamed vegetables for example), with your regular meals will make a big difference in the absorption rate of sugars. So take proteins for lean body mass and a healthy metabolism, but mix the vegetables with the carbs from the point of view of slowing down the absorption of sugars into the body!

Regarding micronutrients common sense is the best approach, but also there are some supplements which you can take which will really help to either improve blood sugar levels or to protect your body from potential degenerative side effects. So let's take a look at them:

Chromium

Chromium has shown some promise in trials as a potential way of improving glucose tolerance levels. In a study which overviewed the results of twenty clinical trials on chromium as a supplement only one demonstrated a noticeable improvement in HB1Ac levels (Altheas MD, Jordan NE, Ludington EA, and Watts JT: Glucose and insulin responses to dietary chromium supplements: a meta-analysis. *Am J Clan Nutria* 76:148-155, 2002) There's not enough research yet to guarantee that chromium helps but it appears at least in this trial to help improve blood sugar control.

43

Zinc

Diabetics lose zinc in their urine although usually they balance things out via zinc absorption in the gastrointestinal tract, but still zinc deficiencies are common. In clinical trials there has been a noted improvement in treating skin ulceration via zinc supplementation (Moravian AD, Faille M, Howler B, Maryniuk M, Wylie-Rosette J

: Selected vitamins and minerals in diabetes. *Diabetes Care* 17:464-479, 1994)

Calcium

In some recent studies it has been noted that calcium and vitamin D help improve immunity modulation and pancreatic insulin secretion (Horlicks MF: Vitamin D deficiency. *N Engle J Med* 357:266-281, 2007*) and (*Rosen CJ: Postmenopausal osteoporosis. *N Engle J Med* 353:595-603, 2005). Calcium and vitamin D are often promoted by the medical community as a way of improving skeletal health, so probably everyone should supplement calcium and vitamin D. Calcium can also be imbibed via milk and other products which are high in calcium but vitamin D tends to be difficult to absorb for most people, so supplementation via pills is a good idea.

Selenium

Selenium shows some potential as an anti-cancer agent, although the evidence is not conclusive. But from the diabetic point of view of diabetics, selenium deficiency tends to be present and when selenium is deficient it result in sugar pangs which makes it difficult for diabetics to keep on track with their diet.

B Vitamins

Diabetics are prone to vitamin B deficiency especially vitamin B12, which can often result in neurological problems. Also the various B vitamins can help to prevent a variety of degenerative health conditions. Folic acid, pyridoxine hydrochloride, and cyanocobalamin when combined, for example, can help to prevent the onset of age-related macular degeneration (AMD) in the eyes.

Vitamin C

Vitamin C has great potential as a way of preventing at atherosclerotic plaque formation; microangiopathy, improving vascular integrity and also it help with wound healing. The only thing to bear in mind with vitamin C is that the body only absorbs 12% of the vitamin C, as the rest is broken down in the gastrointestinal tract. So it's a good idea to take a reasonable dose per day, as in maybe a couple of 500mg pills two or three times a day.

Vitamin E

Vitamin E is a potent antioxidant and possesses good cardio protective properties. In particular vitamin E helps to reduce LDL oxidation and also it helps to stabilize platelet membranes which help to promote cardiovascular health. (Ioannides C, Flatt PRMooradian AD: Micronutrients in diabetes mellitus. *In* Drugs, Diet, and Disease. *Vol.* 2 Ioannides C, Flatt PR, *Eds.* Hemel Hempstead, U.K., Ellis Horwood, 1999, *p.* 183-2)

Alpha-Lipoic Acid

Alpha-lipoic acid (LA) is a potent antioxidant which helps to scavenge free radicals, it chelates transition metal ions, and also it increases cytosolic glutathione and vitamin C levels too. Alpha-lipoic acid helps to prevent the breakdown of beta cells in the pancreas and also it help to protect the body from diabetic neuropathy.

Ok I know that this list of diabetic supplements is as long as my arm, but it's worth taking these supplements as they will help you to both reverse the symptoms of diabetes and also they will protect your health from many possible degenerative health conditions, which is well worth your while in taking them.

46

Exercise and Diabetes

Every medical professional will tell you to exercise on a regular basis so as to help your body to stabilize its sugar levels and this cannot be underestimated. Without some kind of exercise it's almost impossible to reverse diabetic symptoms.

Now how much should you exercise?

Ideally you should perform strenuous exercise, the more strenuous the better. What is important here is that the human body is designed for strenuous exercise and that in our modern daily life, most of us are too sedentry. So this sedentary living makes the body less efficient, which can help to promote diabetes.

So while all exercise is good and I know that many people cannot exercise strenuously, that strenuous exercise, whereby for at least three time a week you push hard for twenty minutes to one hour, will pay of benefits in terms of improving blood sugar control and obviously cardiovascular health as well!

If you cannot exercise strenuously then at least try and perform some exercise, even if it is only a twenty minute walk a day, so as to keep the body moving and getting blood to flow around the organs, as it will help.

Finally before beginning an exercise program do go for a check-up with your doctor, so as to make sure that you are fit enough to exercise. Now this is not necessary if you're just going for a mild walk everyday, but if you are going to take up strenuous exercise, such as weight training, swimming squash, Badminton, soccer etc., then get yourself checked out first, as diabetics are prone to heart problems and you need to check your health out for anything negative here.

For example, high blood pressure is a common side effect of diabetes, now exercise will improve blood pressure levels, but if blood pressure levels are uncontrolled, it will result in a potential for strokes or heart attacks, so something as simple as taking some high blood pressure medication can bring the blood pressure back into line and then taking up exercise and lifestyle changes may well reverse blood pressure over time (for more information on how to treat blood pressure you can check out my book on high blood pressure).

Chapter Four – Super Foods for Diabetes

In the last chapter we looked at supplements which can be used to help improve diabetic symptoms but what about super foods. The following foods naturally reduce blood sugar levels while also protecting the body from the degenerative side effects of diabetes.

Cinnamon/Cardamom/Ginger

Cinnamon

Although often used as an ingredient in tasty cakes cinnamon is an amazing herb with a plethora of great benefits. First off cinnamon is very high in calcium, manganese, iron and vitamin K, Cinnamon is in two types, which are:

· Ceylon cinnamon

· Cassia cinnamon

Cassia cinnamon is the more popular variety of cinnamon, but the healthiest version is Ceylon cinnamon. Cinnamon comes from the cinnamomum tree and cinnamaldehyde is the primary medicinal compound found within cinnamon Just take a look:

- High in antioxidants

- High in anti-inflammatory properties

- Reduces cardiac risk

- Improves insulin sensitivity

- Reduces blood sugar levels in diabetics

- Helps brain health

- Prevents cancer

- Fights bacterial infection

- Fights viral infections

- Protects dental health/ gives fresh breath

- Can prevent /cure candida

- Benefits skin health

- Is a natural preservative/ sweetener

- Fights allergies

Improves Insulin Sensitivity/Anti-Diabetic

Insulin is a vital hormone for the cellular absorption of glucose. However, in some cases the person becomes resistant to insulin, whereby beta cells do not absorb insulin, resulting in the beta cells of the pancreas producing yet more insulin. So with insulin resistance a greater level of insulin is required, so that glucose can be absorbed.

Now insulin resistance is extremely common today, and it seems to come about as a consequence of obesity and lack of exercise. Also, excessive eating appears to upset the hormonal balance and force, as excessive amount of insulin is needed just to absorb the large amount of food. So while a definitive cause of insulin resistance has not been fully determined, probably the lack of exercise, excessive eating and obesity forces the body into working inefficiently.

Insulin resistance is extremely common and most of us probably possess some degree of insulin resistance. So having some insulin resistance is not the end of the world. However, over time it encourages pre-diabetes and pre-diabetes often leads onto to full-blown type 2 diabetes. So insulin resistance can be a slippery slope, which can lead to diabetes.

If you want to avoid insulin resistance, or reduce its severity if you have already developed insulin resistance, then it is important to eat a balanced diet. Don't eat

51

too much processed foods, particularly foods which are very high in simple carbohydrates which force the body to push up insulin levels. So you have to give your stomach and intestines a chance to digest the backlog of food.

Taking a day or two a week and doing some intermittent fasting will help. You don't have to fast for 16 hours, just a mini fast of say 12 – 14 hours, will have a positive effect in that insulin levels will drop and as they do so growth hormone levels will raise. Increased growth hormone, will help fat loss but also it helps to rebalance the hormonal situation, as the body continually flips back and fort between an insulin fat storage state, where human growth hormone (HGH) levels are low and then periods of fasting, whereby the HGH is high and the insulin is low. This is the natural pattern and excessive eating messes this up, while some light intermittent fasting will help to rebalance this.

So for example, maybe you had your last meal at 8pm and you usually have breakfast at 8am, well occasionally hold of and have a brunch at 11am, it's that simply. Also as a final note on this, don't intermittent fast everyday, as eating many meals throughout the day is actually good for blood sugar levels, whereas if you eat say only twice a day, chances are that once again that this can result in insulin resistance, as blood sugar levels keep on fluctuating. Do a small intermittent fast from 1 to 3 days a week and other than that try and eat at least 3, meals a day!

Exercise will also help greatly and of course certain foods will help and once again this is where cinnamon comes in handy!

In a study on the effects of cinnamon on insulin sensitivity, they noted that its chromium and polyphenols promote insulin sensitivity, which in turn reduces fasting blood glucose levels.(Proc Nutr Soc. 2008 Feb;67(1):48-53. doi: 10.1017/S0029665108006010.Chromium and polyphenols from cinnamon improve insulin sensitivity.Anderson RA1).

And in another study, they divided 22 participants into two groups and gave one group 500mg a day of aqueous extract of cinnamon and the second group where given a placebo for 12 weeks. In the cinnamon group they noted a decrease in fasting blood sugar levels, an improvement in blood pressure levels and even an increase in lean body mass(LBM) (LBM denotes how much muscle you have in your body, with age LBM levels drop and this leads onto ill health in old age)!(J Diabetes Sci Technol. 2010 May; 4(3): 685–693. PMCID: PMC2901047Cinnamon: Potential Role in the Prevention of Insulin Resistance, Metabolic Syndrome, and Type 2 DiabetesBolin Qin, M.D., Ph.D.,1,2 Kiran S. Panickar,1 and Richard A. Anderson, Ph.D., C.N.S.1).

Good news for diabetics - cinnamon improves insulin sensitivity 20 fold in a clinical study!

This same research paper goes on to outline how cinnamon, potentiated insulin activity by 20 times more than any other compound, which they examined, also how cinnamon reduces inflammation and how cinnamon kills of cancer cells!

Cinnamon is an amazing herb with great medicinal properties. Also, while researching this and other books I have to read a lot of clinical literature and while other herbs help to reduce fasting blood sugar levels, cinnamon in many different clinical trials, demonstrated the most significant effect on fasting blood sugar levels. As noted earlier a reduction by as much as 29% in the case of individuals who imbibed 6 grams a day!(Diabetes Care. 2003 Dec;26(12):3215-8.Cinnamon improves glucose and lipids of people with type 2 diabetes.Khan A1, Safdar M, Ali Khan MM, Khattak KN, Anderson RA.)

My advice to any diabetic is to make an effort to take various herbs such as ginger and cardamom, but also definitely take cinnamon as it is the most effective blood sugar reducing herb, which you can get your hands on!

Try to take 6 grams a day and keep it up for a least a few weeks, in order to give it a chance to work as herbs take longer to work than allopathic medication. As always I would suggest taking several grams a day, ideally 6 grams, but the most important thing is to take at least a gram or two a day and keep it up, while noting your fasting blood sugar levels regularly!

Cinnamon Reduces Cardiac Risk

Cinnamon also produces a good effect on cardiac health, and noticeably so on diabetic patients, In a study on 60 diabetic patients (5)+9 where split into 3 groups; with dosing varying from 1, 3 or 6 grams of cinnamon per day.

After 40 days the following results where denoted:

Fasting Glucose Serum levels - Reduced by 18 -29% according to dose

Triglycerides – Reduced by 23 -30% according to dose

LDL Cholesterol – Reduced by 7 to 27% according to dose

Total cholesterol levels – Reduced by 12 to 26% according to dose

How to Take Cinnamon

Cinnamon is widely available in health stores and online. You can buy cinnamon as cinnamon rolls, as a tea powder and also as an actual powder, and of course as an oil and as an extract. The most versatile form is as a powder as you can imbibe it in many different ways, such as in a tea or a juice, for instance. While cinnamon is a very tasty food product, on its own it can have a strong taste, so from the point of view of delivering 5 or 6 grams a day, possibly the power mixed in with juice or as a tea is the most efficient way to take cinnamon.

55

Also, from the strength point of view, while cinnamon tea can be tasty, it will lose some of its strength compared with raw unprocessed cinnamon, so with this in mind here is a homemade cinnamon tea recipe.

Cinnamon Tea Recipe

1.   Take a cinnamon stick or 1 tsp. of cinnamon powder

2.   Add to water and boil and then simmer for 10 minutes

3.   Strain and serve

4.   Alternatively to add taste you can mix in another herbal tea

5.   Yet another option is to add in honey and lemon into the mix or even boil some ginger along with the cinnamon and have cinnamon, ginger, lemon and honey tea!

Cinnamon Contraindications

Cinnamon is pretty safe. There are no major side effects, in some cases when using cinnamon for skin some people, suffer from touch dermatitis, but that's rare. As always with any skin product try it out on a small patch first before using it liberally. Other than that a lot of talk is made about how Ceylon cinnamon been superior to cassia cinnamon, but cassia cinnamon also has some benefits and in general while Ceylon is usually more potent, any cinnamon, whichever way you can get it, is going to be a great help.

So cinnamon has a wide variety of uses and usually in the 1 to 6gram mark. For general health 1 gram a day is good and for diabetics a large dose if put to 6grms will be found to be quite useful!

Take 1gram of cinnamon a day for health maintenance and 6 grams a day for relieve from chronic ill health!

This is an amazing result and it's not the only one, as quite a few studies reveal the amazing blood sugar reducing effects of cinnamon. Cinnamon is definitely a must for diabetics and of course the reduction in various types of bad cholesterol. So definitely cinnamon is very good for cardiac health.

Cardamom

We can't write about cinnamon without mentioning cardamom, as cardamom is another popular food ingredient which is famous for its effectiveness as a food additive, but just like cinnamon it's the real deal when it comes to beneficial effects. Let's take a look at its benefits:

- Helps digestion

- Helps bad breath

- Good for oral health

- Detoxifies

- High in antioxidants

- Anti-pathogen

- Fights cold and flu's

- Fights depression

- Reduces blood pressure

- Prevents blood clots

- Anti-inflammatory

- Diuretic

- Hiccup cure

How to Take Cardamom

Cardamom is pretty flexible. It can be added into food for taste, but the cocking process will kill have most of its biota availability, so either drink cardamom tea or for oral health chew cardamom. Another option is to take cardamom as a powder which makes it easy to mix it in with juices and smoothies. In powder form it can easily be both at your nearest health food store and online at a health online retailer.

Regarding dosing we can see a significant reduction with 3 grams a day. So for maintenance take 1 gram a day, if you have a chronic health condition such as cardiovascular issues then go for 2 to 3 grams daily.

For maintenance take 1 gram of cardamom a day and for chronic ill-health take 3 grams a day!

Cardamom Contraindications

Cardamom is really safe, although in some cases liver and brain toxicity can occur, but to get to that level requires vast dudes. In clinical trials put 3 grams a day has been observe end with zero toxicity effects!

Ginger

Ginger is very popular as an ingredient in many tasty recipes, but what most people do not know is that ginger is a fantastic tonic which has the following benefits:

- Ginger strengthens the immune system

- Ginger cures nausea

- Ginger reduces high blood pressure

- Ginger helps to reduce the severity of symptoms associated with osteoarthritis

- Ginger helps to reduce blood sugar levels in diabetics

- Ginger improves digestion

- Ginger reduces bad cholesterol

- Ginger prevents dementia

- Ginger reduces the symptoms of menstrual tension

- Ginger boosts yang energy in the body

- Ginger is a great tonic

Ginger Helps to Reduce Blood Sugar Levels in Diabetics

Like high blood pressure diabetes is in the WHO top 10 of most hazardous diseases. Not that anyone dies from diabetes, but rather they die from complications, which have come about via the long-term degenerative effects of diabetics. So needless to say anything which improves diabetic health is a good thing and the most important factor relating to diabetes is to reduce blood sugar levels. Ginger has been studied and in one trial of 41 participants they noted that over a course of a 12 week period, while taking 2 grams of ginger a day, that the overall average fasting blood sugar levels dropped by 12%. (Iran J Pharm Res. 2015 Winter; 14(1): 131–140.PMCID: PMC4277626The Effects of Ginger on Fasting Blood Sugar, Hemoglobin A1c, Apolipoprotein B, Apolipoprotein A-I and Malondialdehyde in Type 2 Diabetic PatientsNafiseh Khandouzi,a Farzad Shidfar,b,* Asadollah Rajab,c Tayebeh Rahideh,d Payam Hosseini,e and Mohsen Mir Taherif).

This means that a person who has say a borderline diabetic blood sugar level of 140mgdl (7.7 mmol), could see a reduction back down to 125mgdl(6.9mmol), ok not perfect but a lot better for your long-term health than 140/7.7!

The Best Ways to Take Ginger

There are lots of good ways to take ginger supplementation. The easiest way is to take supplements out of a bottle, which is fine, especially since it can be difficult to get enough ginger was raw ginger, is very difficult to take unless you mix it in with a juice or a smoothie. So let's take a look at a few alternatives, as while capsules are fine, raw is always best!

Also regarding dosage around 2 to 3 grams a day is good. If you want to take raw ginger, say in a tea or a juice or a smooth, then it is difficult to know exactly how much you are taking. So as a rule of thumb I would suggest 1 cup or mug of ginger tea for maintenance and 3 cups or mugs a day for anyone who is really drained or removing from chronic ill health.

If you are taking 3 cups a day, of the concentrated "Holistic Super Healthy Ginger Tea" option below then I would recommend only taking this much for 6 weeks at any one time, then take a few weeks at maintenance levels. We have to watch our ying and yang levels, so too much of this herb could burn of nurturing energy at a very high dosage!

Juices and Smoothies: If you want to add ginger into smoothness and juices, it's really easy, simply peel the outer skin from the part of ginger which you intend on taking and then slice off 3 to 5 bits, then throw them in the mix and off you go!

Ginger Tea: Ginger tea is a great option as you can get a real kick out of it. Here are two suggestions:

Traditional Indian Ginger Tea

1.   Mix one cup of milk with one cup of water (this is to make two cups of tea)

2.   Add sugar (if you like sugar) into the mix

3.   Add two teaspoons of tea powder

4.   Add in several slices of ginger (cut and then crush it a little bit so as to get the most out of it)

5.   Boil, simmer and boil simmer gain three times

6.   Strain and serve

Holistic Super Healthy Ginger Tea

1.   Take 2 cups of water (for 2 cups) and add in several slices of ginger (cut and then crush it a little bit so as to get the most out of it)

2.   Boil and leave to simmer for 10 minutes

3.   Squeeze one small lemon or half a medium sized lemon into each cup

4.   Add one to two tablespoons of honey per cup (depending upon taste…ginger tea is very strong so a fair amount of honey is required to take out the sting!)

5.   Strain and pour the ginger water solution into each cup

The advantage with this full blown way to take ginger tea, is that the ginger is so much stronger, because you have let it simmer for a good 10 minutes. So as to know when the concoction is ready, simply waited until the water has taken on a distinct yellowy brown hue.

Anyway the advantage of this concentrated version of ginger tea is that the ginger is very strong, so strong that it should sting your throat a little bit. Also honey and lemon have many great additional benefits.

For general health Indian ginger tea is great, but if you are under the weather and need to pick yourself up or are trying to recover from chronic ill health, then I would suggest going for the more concentrated option!

Contraindications

Ginger is a very safe herb although there are a couple of contraindications.

1.   Ginger slows blood clotting and may adversely affect medications which are designed thin the blood such as 'warfarin'

2.	Ginger reduces blood sugar, to the degree that diabetics should monitor their blood sugar levels, as ginger can cause a pretty severe drop in blood sugar levels in some cases!

3.	Massive doses of concentrated ginger could adversely affect ying energy, but this should not be a problem if you follow the advice given above in the section entitled "The Best Way to Take Ginger"

Aloe Vera

Aloe Vera reduces blood lipids (fats) in the blood, which is an issue for diabetic patients.(Beneficial effects of Aloe vera leaf gel extract on lipid profile status in rats with streptozotocindiabetesS Rajasekaran, K Ravi, K Sivagnanam… - Clinical and …, 2006 - Wiley Online Library).

In another study, on the effectiveness of aloe Vera, they noted a significant reduction in blood glucose levels, within two weeks and triglycerides within 4 weeks.(Antidiabetic activity of Aloe vera L. juice II. Clinical trial in diabetes mellitus patients in combination with glibenclamideN. Bunyapraphatsara1, *, S. Yongchaiyudha1, V. Rungpitarangsi2, O. Chokechaijaroenporn21 Medicinal Plant Information Center, Faculty of Pharmacy, Mahidol University2 Department of Preventive and Social Medicine, Faculty of Medicine Siriraj Hospital, Mahidol University). Furthermore, it helps to decrease swelling and brings about quicker healing of wound injuries (Influence of aloe vera on the healing of dermal wounds in diabetic ratsP Chithra, G.B Sajithlal, Gowri ChandrakasanDepartment of Biochemistry, Central Leather Research Institute, Adyar, Chennai 600 020, IndiaReceived 18 August 1997, Revised 6 October 1997, Accepted 12 October 1997, Available online 4 March 1999), which of
65

course is useful as diabetics have to be careful that they do not develop necrotic tissue.

How to take Aloe Vera for Diabetes:

Two tbsp. of aloe Vera juice per day will make a noticeable improvement.

Bilberry Extract

Bilberries (vaccinium myrtillus) are berries, and like most berries that possess many health benefits which include strengthening blood vessels, improvement of circulation, it prevents cell damage, possibly it might help with retinopathy and also it is good for reducing blood sugar levels.

In particular bilberries contain anthocyanosides, which promote blood vessel strength and which may protect diabetic patients from developing retinal damage 6. Prevention is always better than cure, and diabetics must remember that diabetes isn't simply about high blood sugar, that the high blood sugar levels are damaging to the body and that not only must the blood sugar be lowered but also it is necessary to protect against the side effects.

The side effects of diabetes, in general tend to be heart damage (as a consequence of high triglyceride levels), kidney damage (as a result of cardiovascular damage), nerve damage (which can lead to necrosis), necrosis

66

(which can lead to amputation) and retinopathy. So this quality of bilberries is really important.

Bilberry may have some effect also in lowering blood sugar, but the main benefit of bilberries is as a possible defence against retinopathy.

Since retinopathy is a fairly common occurrence with diabetics, who have diabetes over a period of many years, it makes sense to take bilberries as a possible preventative measure, and also bilberries are really tasty, so it's all win!

The other important side effect, of bilberries, is on blood circulation and vascular health, with research suggesting that bilberries possess vascular protective qualities.7 Lack of good blood circulation and arterial damage, in diabetics, result in a crescendo of negative side effects. Bilberries will help to protect the cardiovascular system, which is really helpful!

How to take Bilberries for Diabetes:

Approximately 20 to 60grams a day produce a good result, and up to 160mg of bilberry extract have been taken by people who have retinopathy with some promising results.8

Bilberry extract can be found in capsules or powder. Take capsules as per grams suggested, of bilberry recommended per day. As a powder it, can be mixed with food or drinks. Also, bilberries can be acquired as crushed bilberries, which once again can be mixed with foods. This is ideal for making shakes, or even for mixing with ice cream or whipped cream to make a really tasty and healthy snack!

Bilberry Tea:

If you can get your hands on bilberry leaves, it is possible to make a delicious bilberry tea.

1.   Boil water and add in 1 gram, which are 2 the spoonful's of chopped dried bilberry leaves.

2.   Leave too steep for 10 minutes.

3.   Filter and serve.

Bilberry Contraindications:

•   Bilberry may make diabetic medicine over effective, consequently diabetics need to check their sugar levels regular, when they start to take bilberry, and adjust the level of medications which they take accordingly.

•   Medications which slow blood clotting (anticoagulant / antiplatelet drugs) are made more effective by bilberry intake. Since bilberries already slow down blood clotting, the combination of bilberries with blood clotting medication may result in excessive bleeding and bruising. Examples of these

68

drugs include clopidogrel (Plavix), ibuprofen (Advil, Motrin, others) and warfarin.

Fenugreek

Fenugreek is an annual plant, in the family Fabaceae, and is widely used as a food ingredient in Asian foods, such as curries and other Indian recipes.

Fenugreek also possess a wide variety of health benefits, which includes the ability of reduce cholesterol, protect the heart, relives constipation, benefits the kidneys and also helps to relieve diabetic symptoms.

Fenugreek seed (trigonella foenum graecum) are high in soluble fibre, which aids blood sugar control as it slows down the absorption of carbohydrates.

In a study on fenugreek, they took 25 patients, splitting them into two groups, a placebo group and a fenugreek group. They gave the fenugreek group 1gram a day of fenugreek, and after two months the fenugreek group saw a noticeable reduction in blood sugar levels, as well as an improvement in insulin senility and a decrease in unhealthy cholesterol levels.(Effect of Trigonella foenum-graecum (fenugreek) seeds on glycaemic control and insulin resistance in type 2 diabetes mellitus: a double blind placebo controlled study.(PMID:11868855)Gupta A ,

Gupta R , Lal BJaipur Diabetes and Research Centre.The Journal of the Association of Physicians of India [2001, 49:1057-1061]).

How to take Fenugreek:

On scientific experiments, fenugreek has been taken anywhere from 2 grams to 100 grams per day. So this is quite a variance. The best advice is to take a smallish dosage of fenugreek, once and twice a day, and see how it goes and adjust if necessary.

Fenugreek seeds are readily available in stores as a culinary food extract. It can come as seeds and as powders and pastes.

Roasted Fenugreek: Fenugreek seeds can be roasted and added into curries.

Fenugreek Powders and Pastes: Fenugreek can be added into food as a powder or as a paste.

Fenugreek tea:

1.   Boil water.

2.   Add in 2tbsp of fenugreek leaves.

3.   Leave to simmer for 10 minutes.

4.   Strain and serve.

Fenugreek Contraindications:

•   Fenugreek seeds may make diabetic medications more effective, consequently diabetics should keep an eye on their medications and reduce as need be so as to avoid low blood sugar levels.

•   Medications which slow blood clotting (anticoagulant / antiplatelet drugs) are made more effective by fenugreek intake. Since fenugreek already slow down blood clotting, the combination of fenugreek with blood clotting medication may result in excessive bleeding and bruising. Examples of these drugs include clopidogrel (plavix), ibuprofen (advil, motrin, others) and warfarin.

Evening Primrose Oil

Evening Primrose Oil is a great supplement , which works well on menopausal symptoms, osteoporosis care, skincare, anti-inflammatory properties and it's good for cardiovascular health, and of course nerve health!

Evening Primrose Oil contains gamma linoleic acid, which helps in repairing damaged nerve cells. In clinical trials, when they gave 480mg of Evening Primrose Oil, for a period of one year, the participants demonstrated signs of nerve repair. (. Keen H, Payan J, Allawi J, et al. Treatment of diabetic neuropathy with gamma-linolenic acid. The gamma-Linolenic Acid Multicenter Trial Group. Diabetes Care. 1993;16:8-15.abstract)

This is very helpful for diabetics, as many diabetics suffer nerve damage, especially to the feet and end up getting cuts, which become gangrenous and then this leads onto severe problems, which can end up with amputation of the lower limbs!

So definitely Evening Primrose Oil is a must for any diabetic patient who wants to prevent nerve damage!

Chapter Five – Chinese Medicine/ Acupressure/Hatha Yoga/Taoist Yoga & Pranayama

So far we have looked at diabetes from a western allopathic perspective. We have looked at lifestyle, diet, exercises and of course super foods which can all help you to gain better control of your diabetes or prediabetes. But we have as yet to look at oriental healthcare and what it has to offer.

In this chapter we shall take a look at Chinese medicine and Indian yoga techniques. Looking first at Traditional Chinese Medicine (TCM), it puts forward the theory that everything is energy (Qi… pronounced as Chi) and that this can further be broke down into ying (nurturing energy) and yang (active energy). From a Chinese medical perspective there is no difference between objects and energy, for example. The chair which you are sitting on and the thoughts in your head are all Qi energy, the only difference been the quality of energy.

Now this might sound outlandish but think again, for with Chinese medicine there is no duality, rather everything is a spectrum, a continuum as it where!

Now how this helps us in dealing with ill health is that it prevents over categorisation from taking place. Often with allopathic medicine there is a tendency to categorise everything from a labelling point of view, which concludes that diabetes is a disease, people with diabetes are patients, and you have to live with diabetes and so on. While this is true to a degree, it tends to reduce diabetes and all forms of ill-health into a bunch of symptoms, which require a bunch of drugs to treat them!

Now Chinese medicine is interested in the energetic dimension, so that while it might be true that diabetes is a mix of genetics and lifestyle, in most cases, it's also true from a TCM perspective that there are energetic imbalances which lie behind ill health. Often western medicine takes a very narrow perspective which makes recovery a challenge, rather its focus on treating symptoms, whereas the approach suggested by TCM allows for a recovery from ill health, because it sees ill-health as an energetic imbalance.

In Traditional Chinese Medicine the organs of the body are seen as having a symbolic effect on health. So for example, diabetes can be tracked back to spleen, kidney and liver imbalances. Now this does not refer back to the functions of the actual organs, rather these are labels which are placed upon the organs describing an energetic role in the body. We must remember that the ancient Chinese medical practitioners did not know much about how the organs actually worked, but they had a great understanding as to how energy moved around the body. They then labelled these energies according to organs.

Anyway from a TCM perspective, diabetes begins as a deficiency, which over time results in the body not been able to balance the control of sugars in the body. Systems like acupuncture, homeopathy and Ayurveda medicine can in some cases make a big impact in improving blood sugar control and are well worth considering, if you want to reverse your diabetes. It's unlikely that anyone of these therapies will make for a cure of diabetes, but they might well help to rebalance the energetic balance in your body, which in turn may help to reverse your diabetes!

The Indian system of hatha yoga also bases its action according to the idea of energetic dynamics within the human body. In hatha yoga they talk about pranic energy and prana instead of Qi, but what their actually talking about is once again Qi energy (which they called prana) and how to make the body balance it's inner energetic dynamics.

So how then can we use Chinese medicine and Hatha yoga in our daily life's so as to improve the energetic balance within our bodies?

From a TCM perspective the three organs which tend to be out of balance are:

Spleen – Which controls the flow of fluids in the body, is responsible for strength in the limbs and is easily burnt off by either thinking too much, doing too much activity or a poor diet.

Kidney – As an energy kidney energy is responsible for growth and reproduction in the body. Kidney energetic imbalances result in a deep seated weakness in the body including weak knees, a weak lower back, feeling cold and weak. Often spleen deficiency will lead onto kidney deficiency.

Liver – As energy the liver is responsible for the flow of energy in the body and also it rules the muscles and tendons in the body. The liver energy must run smoothly for the proper operation of the body.

In Chinese medicine these energies can be either deficient (too little), stagnant (not moving) or excess (too much). Diabetes will often begin as a deficiency and over time it will eat away at the body making it weaver over time, producing symptoms of deficiency in some organs and symptoms of stagnation or excess in another.

From a TCM perspective we have to bring excess energy down, release stagnant energy and bring up deficient energy. Through the human body are lines of energy, which are known as meridians and these meridians are interspaced with nodal points of concentrated energy, which are known as points. By performing either acupressure or reflexology on these points on a daily basis, we can go a long way towards restoring the energetic balcony in the body.

Hand and Foot Acupressure Points

Acupressure is really underrated but it can transform your health!

It's very simple really, all you have to do is to take a few minutes out to press hard on an acupressure point and this point will stimulate this particular organ (we are speaking about energetic organs here, so they are metaphorical in character).

So what points should you stimulate to help reverse diabetes?

Here they are:

- Spleen

- Kidneys

- Liver

- Stomach

- Intestine

- Gall Bladder

- Urinary

- Lung

- Heart

- Pancreas

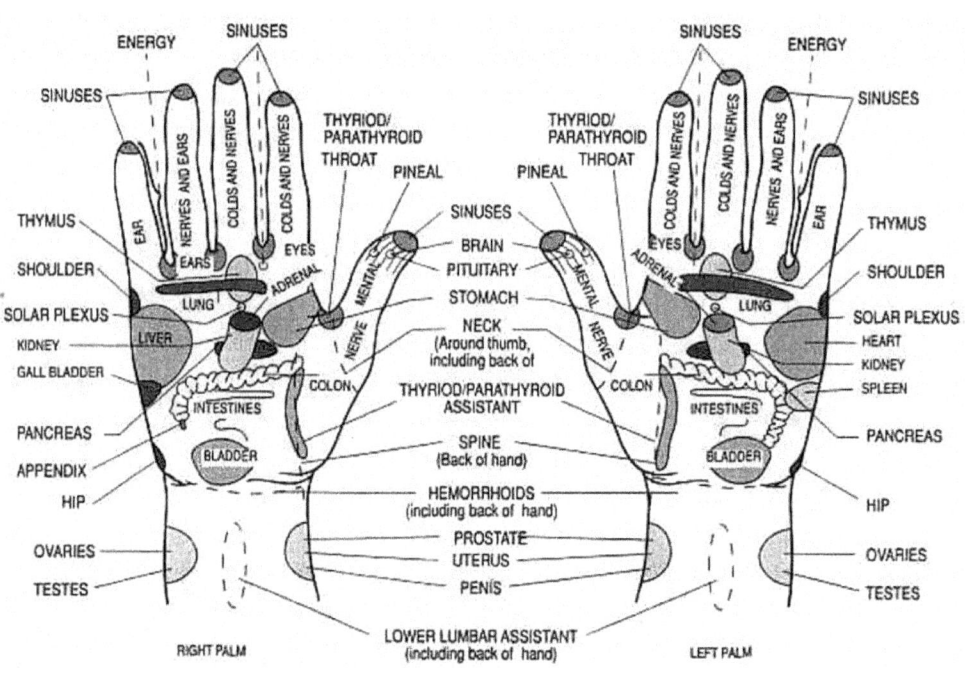

ENERGY   SINUSES   SINUSES   ENERGY

SINUSES   SINUSES

NERVES AND EARS   COLDS AND NERVES   COLDS AND NERVES   NERVES AND EARS

THYRIOD/PARATHYROID   THYRIOD/PARATHYROID
THROAT   THROAT
PINEAL   PINEAL

THYMUS   EAR   EYES   THYMUS

SINUSES

BRAIN

PITUITARY

SHOULDER   EARS   ADRENAL   ADRENAL   SHOULDER
                    LUNG   MENTAL STOMACH MENTAL   LUNG
SOLAR PLEXUS   NERVE   NERVE   SOLAR PLEXUS

NECK
(Around thumb,
including back of

KIDNEY   LIVER   HEART
GALL BLADDER   COLON   COLON   KIDNEY
                       INTESTINES   THYRIOD/PARATHYROID   INTESTINES   SPLEEN
                                   ASSISTANT

PANCREAS   BLADDER   SPINE   BLADDER   PANCREAS
APPENDIX   (Back of hand)
HIP   HEMORRHOIDS   HIP
                             (including back of hand)

OVARIES   PROSTATE   OVARIES
                             UTERUS
TESTES   PENIS   TESTES

LOWER LUMBAR ASSISTANT
(including back of hand)

RIGHT PALM   LEFT PALM

78

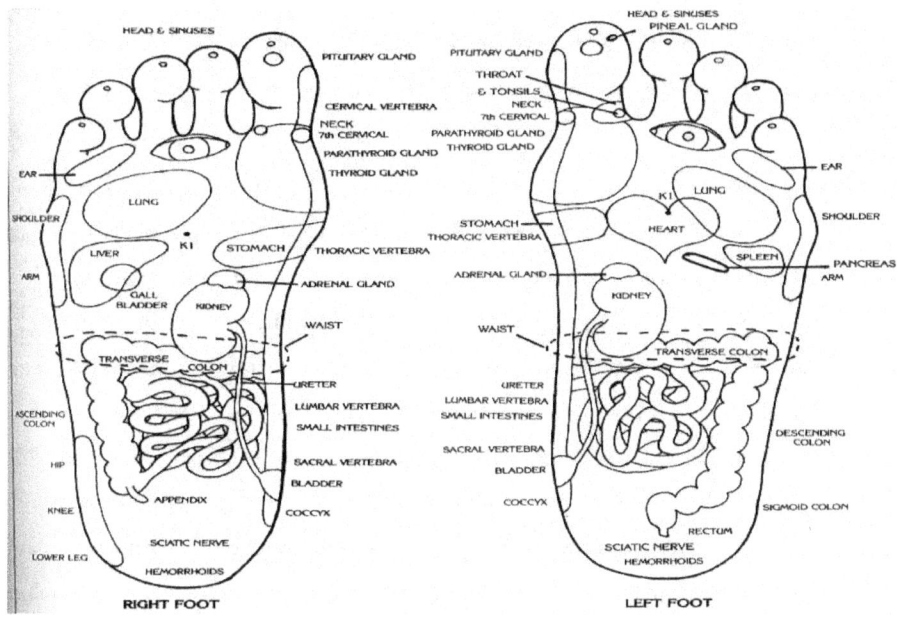

RIGHT FOOT   LEFT FOOT

So the principle is simple, take a point and press it hard until it hurts a little and hold it for a couple of minutes and then move into the next point and so on. The points listed above if massaged regularly will gently bring up the energy levels in these organs. Over time if you are regular the subtle Qi energy through the body will start to balance out.

Also you can use some implements to help. For example you can get an acupressure hand tool whereby it saves you having to squeeze with your fingers, rather you take this device and press with it and let it do the squeezing. You can also use hand rollers and foot reflexology mats. Shop around in health stores or online and use what works for you. The main point is to massage either your hands and /or feet every day. Like I noted earlier, acupressure is really underestimated as it works, just squeeze your hands and feet and keep it up.

Traditional Chinese Medicine (TCM) can often confuse people, because it uses a funny terminology and many of its concepts, including the theory of Qi, ying and yang and so on. But another take on it which might help you to get your head around it, is that acupressure moves the blood, not just in your hands and feet but all over your body. These subtle energy channels, boost energy levels but also they boost blood flow to do these organs, and a healthy organ is an organ which is flushed with fresh blood, which in turn helps the body to get rid of waste products, take new nutrients into the cells and regenerate that particular organ. So regular acupressure practice, along with Hatha yoga and Taoist yoga, helps to heal the body, so just try it out!

Taoist Yoga

Taoist yoga is a phrase which become popularised for describing oriental energetic exercises, which are similar in their function to hatha yoga exercises. Although there is one difference in that with Taoist yoga the exercises are far easier to perform.

The exercises which follow are common popular Taoist exercises which will greatly help to restore the health and balance within your body. Remember things like diet, exercise and even taking supplements only help to relieve symptoms, but with herbs and oriental energetic exercises, it is possible to rebalance the inner energetics of the body over time. It won't happen in one day and certainly once undermined its nearly impossible to bring the body back to its prime level of functioning, but certainly in many cases a great improvement, not only in symptoms alleviation, but also in general health and wellbeing can and will take place, if you practice these exercises diligently every day!

The Crane, the Turtle and the Solar Plexus Exercises

If you Google these exercise, a few options will come up and most of them are difficult to perform. However, exercises of the same name but which are easy to perform, and at the same time are very beneficial, have already been popularised back in the early 1980's by Stephen T Chang and his famous books on Taoist healing techniques. I like these particular variations because of their simplicity and effectiveness. There are lots of interesting exercises, out there, but which are difficult to perform, and really it's not necessary to wrap your legs around your head, in order to heal your body. Rather, many exercises which originate from Taoist healing systems are very easy to perform and should be popularised once again because they really are that good.

Crane

Starting with the Crane, it is named in deference to the crane bird which sucks its abdomen in towards its back bone when standing. A simple variation of this is to simply lie on your back and breath. Breath out while trying to suck your navel back in towards your spine, then breath in and literarily fill up your abdomen until it bloats outward, almost as if it's about to burst. Sucking ones abdomen inwards massages the stomach and intestines, while breathing very deeply into the abdomen charges the stomach with air. Young babies practice abdominal breathing, whilst most adults perform superficial breathing via the top of their lungs; breathing from the abdomen is the natural way to breath. Filling the abdomen first and then the lungs results in a really deep and beneficial breath.

Benefits

The crane has several benefits, which includes the following:

- Strengthening the stomach (which aids digestion and energy production)
- Massaging the intestines (which aids digestion and energy production and prevents constipation)
- Deep breathing stimulates the nervous system and oxygenates the blood (which in turn reduces blood pressure)
- Deep breathing combined with deep exhalations extract toxins from the blood
- Deep inhalations combined with deep exhalations, carried out with conscious intent promotes yang energy (active energy) in the body.

Technique

1. Lie down.
2. Breath out, while sucking in your abdomen, focus upon the navel retracting towards the spinal cord. Go as far as is comfortable and then

82

squeeze slightly. This process can then be enhanced by pressing gently downwards, with the palms of your hands.

3. When fully exhaled immediately inhale, by breathing into the abdomen and filling up your belly until it fills like its ready to explode. At this stage the breath will naturally fill the lungs from the lower position. Hold for a few seconds and then exhale once again.

4. Repeat this process of exhalation followed by deep inhalation and continue for about five minutes in total.

It is important, with this exercise to carry it out gently. Do not force, rather gently exhale and gently inhale. Also, there is a good chance that some slight discomfort will be felt during the exhalation. This is fine, the reason for this, is because most of us have backed up faeces, within our intestines. Which is a common, side effect of highly processed foods, and lack of fibre in our diet. Keep with the program and gently massage the lower intestines, by gently squeezing (but not forcing) the lower intestines.

With this exercise, blood will gently seep into the microvilli of the lower intestines, which in turn will aid digestion and health in general.

What has this exercise got to do with high blood pressure?

This is a great exercise for building up the two most important organs of the body, from the point of view of health and vitality. A strong stomach will break down food efficiently, while strong clean intestines will effectively absorb nutrients into the body. The effect of these two organs been boosted is an

improved immune system, higher vitality levels and improved yang (active)
energy, which in turn helps to balance blood pressure naturally.

The Solar Plexus Exercise

Like Stephen T Chang, I am a great believer in this exercise, although the way I
do it differs considerable from his method. The way I recommend doing this
exercise is twofold, it involves massaging the solar plexus and also using
visualisation exercises.

From a nervous point of view, the solar plexus is a major nerve group, within the
body. The solar plexus is found at the base of the sternum. Lie down and poke
this area with your finger, when a sudden stabbing pain is felt, then bingo! This is
the solar plexus. From a TCM point of view, the solar plexus represents the
emotional brain, while the physical brain is simply a computing machine.
Whenever we feel upset or overwhelmed, we feel discomfort in the solar plexus.
Stage nerves, when we have to step up and speak in front of others and feeling
nauseous when facing an interview, are obvious examples of an overwhelmed
solar plexus. Also, in the case of kids, often their stomach aches are actually
caused by emotional overwhelming feelings, in the solar plexus and massaging
will often help greatly.

84

The solar plexus is really important, because our bodies are designed for a far simpler era, consequently, we often feel overwhelmed because we are designed for simple living.

Solar plexus exercises will greatly help to calm down anxious feelings and obviously this will help blood pressure levels because of the feelings of rejuvenation which come from this exercise, since often high blood pressure levels are created by tension and feelings of being overwhelmed. So this is a great deep relaxation exercise.

Technique

1. Lie down.
2. Locate the solar plexus and begin massaging it in a clockwise manner. This is particularly useful when feeling hurt feelings and anxious feelings. If general fatigue is felt, but emotions are not disturbed then just jump ahead to the next stage.
3. Hold both hands either side of the solar plexus and then visualise divine white light (or egg yolk yellow, if you like – as this is the astral colour of the solar plexus chakra) gently filling the solar plexus.
4. Maintain this position and occasionally remind oneself of the light. Continue for five to fifteen minutes.

Also, if you like soft music can be played along while this gently recharging process is taking place.

Turtle

The turtle is a simple exercise, yet it is a great way to relax the neck and shoulders, which in turn brings about relaxation and consequently this de-stressing effect promotes relief of high blood pressure.

Benefits

1. Stretches the spine.
2. Relaxes the shoulders and neck.
3. Boosts the thyroid and parathyroid.
4. Boosts the metabolism.
5. Boosts inner energy delivery within the body.

Technique

1. Sit (cross legged or on a chair).
2. Bring your chin down to your chest and slowly inhale. The neck will feel slightly stretched while the shoulders will relax deeply.
3. Slowly lift the head upwards and backwards, until the back of the head touched the atlas joint, at the back of the neck. Exhale while doing so, this time the throat will feel stretched.
4. Repeat twelve times, but do not strain.

Contraindications

In general this is a very safe exercise but do bear in mind that for someone who suffers from serious neck injuries or scoliosis, for example, might feel pain and it might be damaging. So obviously, use your common sense. No discomfit should be felt either during or after this exercise. If any discomfort if felt, do stop immediately!

Hatha Yoga

Just like Taoist yoga, Hatha yoga can help to rebalance the inner energetics of the body over a period of time. Hatha yoga postures (asanas) tend to be difficult to perform but what follows are some of the easier ones which will help to reverse your diabetes.

Savasanna

Many people don't know how to relax and relaxation is a first step towards regaining your health. What follows is a quick outline of a really simple hatha yoga asana, which is savasanna (relaxed poise). If you relax easily then you can skip it, but if you struggle to relax then give this a try as relaxation is the foundation upon which we can rebuild our health. When we relax our bodies it provides our bodies with the inner resources required to bringing about the healing process.

Savasanna, otherwise known as the corpse pose, is without doubt the easiest hatha yoga pose, which can be performed. In Savasanna, the practitioner simply lies on their back with their legs and arms stretched outward, as if in a five star formation. While, it is very simple, do not underestimate its effectiveness, as it is designed to greatly reduce physical stress and its effect on blood pressure levels is easily noted, as blood pressure always ties into physical stress levels.

1. Lie on your back with arms and legs outstretch at a 45 degree angle.
2. Maintain hands in an open upturned pose.
3. Relax and breathe deeply.
4. Stay in this position for five to ten minutes

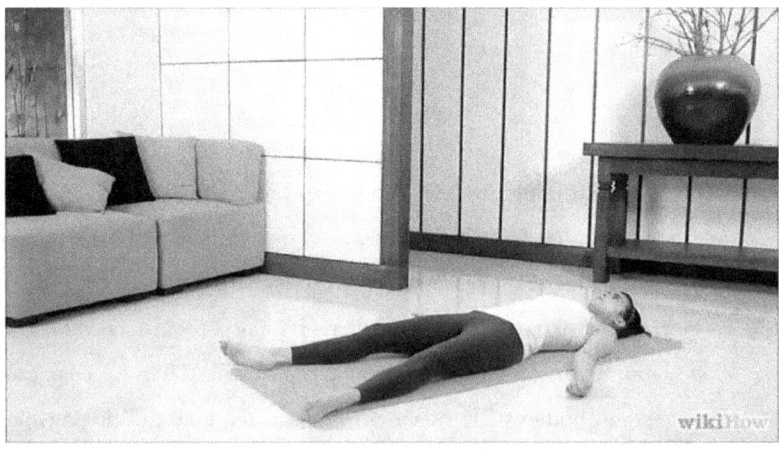

Uddiyana Bandha

Uddiyna bandha (flying upward) is a fairly simple hatha yoga asana which is normally seen as a purification exercise. However, it is also very good at strengthening the inner body, which is a big help for diabetics.

The procedure in uddiyana bandha simple involves standing up and hunching over with your hands pressed firmly on your thighs just above your knees. You then breath out and when all the air is out suck in your abdomen imagining as if their where a cord connecting your belly button to your backbone and pull in as far as you can, hold for a second and then let go.

This is the basic procedure although there are many variations. The most popular variations are usually based on very quick movements of the abdomen, whereby the abdomen is sucked in and out very quickly, the idea been to do this ten times, which is one round, and then rest for a second or two while you catch a couple of breath send repeat again. Starting of with one round and day and working up potentially to many dozens of rounds.

Personally I prefer a slower approach to this exercises, for unless you re fairly skinny with very good abdominal strength it will be difficult to really feel this exercise working, also it can be difficult to get enough air in between rounds, as you do not breath during the round. So once again unless your fit, slim and have strong abs chances are that breathing will be a strain. So for ordinary individuals, like myself for example, I recommend a slower approach whereby you suck in your abdomen and hold for a second rather than immediately repasting the exercise, let UT your stomach, breath in again and out again and then once more suck in your abdomen and hold for a second. This is a far lower process, but you can really feel it working even if you're not much if a hatha yogi.

In particular from an energetic point of view what we are after is an energetic boost. Now uddiyna has many benefits simply because when we suck in our abs it stimulates blood flow into the midsection thus heeling digestion and boosting pancreatic functioning, but we can also get a boost from energetic locks which are known as band has. In this exercise if we do it right we can get an epiglottis (the flap of flesh in the back of our throat) lock and also an anal (as in anus in our bottom) lock, When we suck in tightly wehile focused on sealing the anus and epiglottis we will feel our throat close and also our anus lift up. Bellevue it or not this creates a terrific energetic boost for the body.

Variation on Uddiyana Bandha

Also uddiynaa bandha can be difficult to perform if your overweight so a couple of simple variations here are to either lie back down on the floor or the bed or a mat or whatever, then fold your legs as if you were sitting with your leg crossed but instead you are lying down with your legs crossed. This posture is known as the poise of the fish. Anyway it will naturally bring about a sucking in of the stomach, which will help to make this exercise easier.

90

Yet another variation is to sit on all fours like a dog when it stands and perform uddiynaa in this position, which is particularly good for prom opting epiglottis and anal bandhas!

Uddinyana bandha is an exercise which can be performed every day and over time your abdominal muscles will become stronger and more toned which will help you posture and also it will help to make you look slimmer, but more importantly it will go a long way towards replenishing the organs of the lower trunk, which in turn will help the body to produce more insulin naturally!

Paschimottanasana (Forward Bend Pose)

Paschimottanasana, is a very simple yet effective asana (posture). It can be difficult to perform it to its full extent, but do not worry if you find yourself only able to complete half the stretch, as over time flexibility will increase. The important thing is to give the legs and back a good stretch. In the process of doing so blood flow to the middle of the body will increase and in particular the lower back and hamstrings.

Regardless how deep you get into the posture, do hold the final position for a few seconds in order to allow the increased blood flow to do its work.

Benefits:

- Relieves blood pressure
- Sooths anxiety
- Promotes calmness
- Relaxes nerves
- Reduces fatigue
- Reduces sinusitis
- Good for ovaries and uterus
- Good for kidneys and liver
- Good for spinal health
- Relieves insomnia
- Improves digestion

Technique

1. Sit on the floor with legs outstretched.
2. Ease arms directly above the head.
3. Stretch the hands and arms downwards towards the toes. If possible clasp the soles of the feet and hold this stretch for five seconds. If this is not possible then simply stretch to whatever is comfortable for you.
4. Release and once again sit upright
5. Repeat eight times.

Contraindications:

- Do not practice in case of a herniated disc.
- It might not be appropriate for some pregnant ladies.

- Avoid if suffering from hip problems
- Avoid if suffering from sciatica.

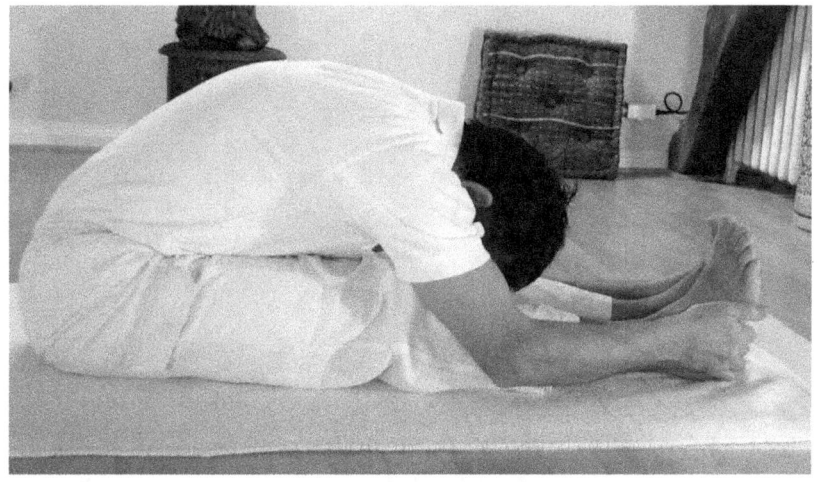

Photo Courtesy of Joseph RENGER

(https://commons.wikimedia.org/wiki/File:Paschimottanasana.jpg#filelinks)

Shashankasana (hare pose) and Balasana Pose (Pose of a Child)

Both of these are simple poses whereby the practitioner sits on their knees. In the case of balasana, the body is folded and the arms rest at ones side, whereas with shashankasana, the arms are outstretched in front.

Benefits:

Both poses have similar benefits to Paschimottanasana, in that they involve the bending forward of the body, which stimulates the spine and inner organs. Also, all of these postures are extremely relaxing, and this is the main thing, from the point of view of reducing blood pressure levels. The benefits come from increased blood flow and energetic flow via the reflow of panic energy.

Shashankasana provides a better stretch than balasana, so really it's a case of trying both and seeing which one works best for you.

Techniques

1. Sit on your knees.
2. In balasana, rest the weight of your upper body upon your legs, whereby the chest rests on the thighs and let the head rest on the floor, while the arms are on the sides.
3. In the case so shashankasana, begin the same but instead of placing arms on your side, stretch them out in front instead.
4. Hold the position for a comfortable time period. Stat with thirty seconds and work up to two minutes. Don't worry about repetitions, rather make yourself comfortable and stay there while comfortable, then sit back up again then resume after a few seconds. In total two or three repetitions, with extended time periods where the pose is held, is ideal.

SHASHANKASANA

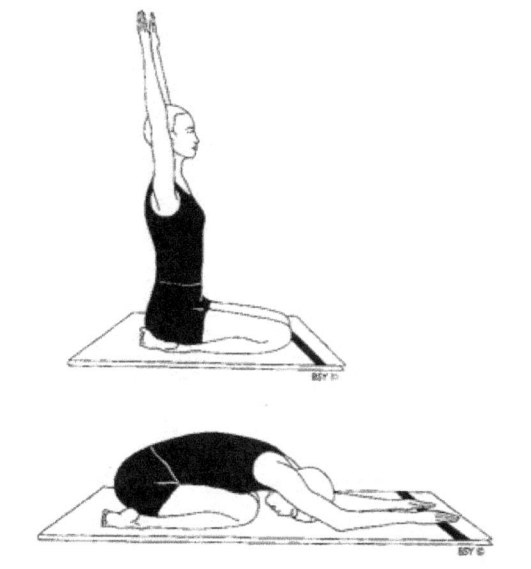

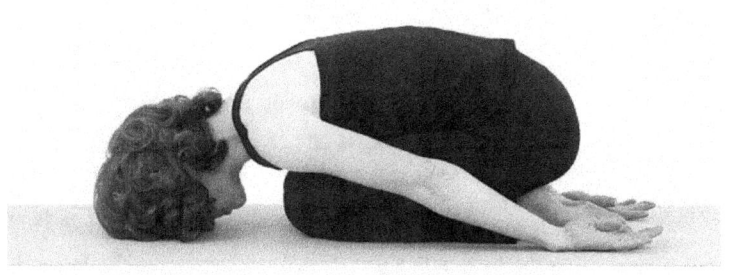

Photo Courtesy of https://vikasacharya.wordpress.com/2015/06/13/how-the-yoga-asana-helps-in-fertility/

Dhanurasana (Bow pose)

Benefit:

It improves Improves the functioning of pancreas and intestines, which in turn helps to in control blood sugar levels. The intestines will work more effectively as a result of these exercises as too will the liver, and the pancreas beta cells are made.

Method:

1. Lie on your stomach and with your arms by the side of your body.

2. Bend your knees and grab your ankles.

3. Breathing in, pull your ankles towards your body while at the same time lifting up your chest and keeping your chine pointing forwards and a little upwards. By pulling on your ankles while lifting up your chest your upper torso will automatically go upwards as the arms and legs act as levers pulling up the body.

4. Try and maintain this poise for a few seconds, which might be difficult at first as it is strenuous and will give the muscles of the legs, arms and back a good workout. You know this poise is working when you feel your body is body is taut like a bow.

5. After a few seconds relax and drop back down to the floor. Take a few breath and repeat several times.

An Important Note on Performing Yoga Asanas

Yoga asanas are incredibly helpful, at rebalancing the body, and as a consequence of this they are an effective way to heal oneself. However, for anyone who has not tried hatha yoga before, it can come as a real shock when exercises, which appear easy to perform, turn out to be especially challenging. The thing to remember, with hatha yoga postures, is that there is a presumption that the practitioner is already in good health!

It must be remembered, that for many thousands of years most people where physically active and hence had fairly good flexibility levels. The original creators of hatha yoga, developed these postures, at a time, when the general populace where busy working in physical jobs and so already had well-toned, flexible physiques. Also, back in ancient India most people did not use chairs, indeed chairs are a recent feature of Indian life, and many younger Indians still like to sit on the floor rather than the chair. Chairs, while been a great invention, limit the range of hip motion and consequently people who sit on chairs a lot, have restricted hip mobility.

All of these factors add up to make even the most basic yoga asanas, difficult for many people to perform today. The exercises, listed above, have been picked because of their relative ease, but still some degree of difficulty might initially be felt, particularly in physically heavier people and older people.

Do not worry, if for now, you cannot complete these poses. The traditional approach, to mastering yoga asanas, is to begin slowly and do the best you can without straining. Practice daily and observe over time an increase in flexibility. The key is to practice daily and even the more difficult poses can be mastered. Stick with it for a few weeks, and the poses mentioned above will become far more doable, within a few weeks.

Also, perform the asanas slowly and deliberately. Trying to concentrate, on the movement and focus on good form, these are not western calisthenics, which need to be rushed through in order to get the burn. Rather they need to be applied slowly and with complete awareness, this will give the internal organs the necessary gentle message, which is necessary in order to see good, progressive and safe results!

Pranayama

Pranayama is the name giving to the Indian system of breathing exercises which along with hatha yoga are aimed at helping to boost our health. Now the more advanced pranayama's can be potentially dangerous and should not be practiced without the help of a trained pranayama teacher, but there are some basic pranayama's, which we can use to help promote a healing effect in our bodies.

Here are a few of the easier and safer pranayama's which you can perform so as to help reverse your diabetes.

Anulum Vilum

Benefits of Pranayama Anulom Vilom

1. Improved blood circulation
2. Mind calmness
3. It helps to prevent cardiac health problems
4. It helps to relax the body
5. It cleanses and strengthens the nervous system
6. It improves concentration
7. It can help to prevent diabetes and it can also help to reverse the condition to some degree
8. It can help to remove blockages in the arteries
9. It improves the skin quality
10. It improves the efficiency of the lungs
11. It can help to relieve high blood pressure..
12. It cans relief asthma sinusitis and headaches.

Method:

1. Sit comfortably on the floor with your legs crossed or if you can't cross your legs then simply sit in your chair.

2. Now close the right nostril with right thumb and breathe in from left nostril. Then close the left nostril with middle and ring fingers and breathe out from the right nostril.

3. Breathe in deeply with right nostril and then again close the right nostril and breathe out deeply once more with the left nostril.

4. Repeat 50 times on each side.

Precaution

1. Pregnant women should not practice anulom vilom.

2. Always practice on an empty stomach.

3. Practice 4-5 hours after having food.

Bhastrika (Bellows Breath)

This exercise is known as the bellows exercise because we breathe in and out quickly as if our lungs where a bellows. It is a very powerful exercise, but also it can be a dangerous exercise for people who are suffering from heart and lung problems. It is possible for a person who has lung or heart problems to perform bhastrika, but they have to be very careful and start of easily and see if it works for them and if not then drop it.

Anyway most people get a great health boost from bhastrika but start of gentle and see how it goes!

Benefits of Bhastrika Pranayama

1. Improved blood circulation
2. Prevents heart related problems
3. Relaxes body and mind
4. Improves concentration.
5. It strengthens the lungs.
6. Relives stress and hypertension.
7. Helps fight obesity
8. Improves symptoms of arthritis.
9. Cures throat infections.
10. Improves lagging appetite.
11. Can help improve asthma
12. Helps relieve gastric problems
13. Improves blood sugar control

Method

1. Sit comfortably on the floor with your legs crossed or if you can't cross your legs then simply sit in your chair.
2. Breathe in forcefully and immediately breathe out forcefully.

3. The tempo of breathing can be slow, moderate or extremely fast. Start of slow and see how it feels and increase speed over time. If you have ling or heart problems stay with a slow steady breathing process

4. Do this for 2 min to 5 minutes in one sting for a maximum of two times per day.

Precautions

This can be dangerous for people with heart and lung problems. If you have these problems then start of slow and see how it goes, if you feel any stress then stop immediate, but for many people if they practice gently,works really well at improving the overall health and wellbeing of the body, because it stimulates oxygenated blood flow.

Also, some people get carried away with bhastrika and shake their torsos in a crazy way for a long period of time, which can actually end up creating damage to their internal organs!

So don't do anything silly, bhastrika is a great exercise and can help your diabetes but be careful it is a powerful exercise and it is better to perform it gently and carefully!

Chapter Six – Putting Everything Together

In this book we have looked at a variety of strategies which you can use to help to reverse your diabetes. As outlined in detail in part one, since 8% of the world's population suffers with diabetes, the voracity of the complaint will vary from one person to another. Technically speaking it is impossible to be cured from full blown diabetes (where there is significant damage to the beta cells in the pancreas) without undergoing a miracle. So when people are talking about reversing diabetes, this really only occur in prediabetes whereby the body is suffering from insulin resistance but little or no damage has occurred to the beta cells as of yet. Still for anyone who has full blown diabetes. it may not be possible to reverse the organic damage but it is possible to reverse many of the symptoms. In many cases it is possible to become symptom free, although if you stop the restorative measures and resume a sedentary lifestyle with a junk food diet, the diabetes will kick off again. In some more severe cases of diabetes, some symptoms will still remain, but even so it's worth trying your best to reverse at least some of the symptoms of diabetes!

I know that all of this sounds complicated and this is because it is complicated. Diabetes is not a disease rather it is a health condition, which has a wide variety of symptoms and levels of intensity. It's simply not possible for every diabetic person to reverse their diabetes, but on the other hand it is far easier to reverse many of the symptoms of diabetes, than one may realise at first. It is possible to improve your diabetic symptoms, reverse some altogether and prevent many of the long-term degenerative side effects along the way, and this goes for every diabetic, whereas for others a complete reversal can take place in some of the more moderate cases. Either way it makes sense to do everything which you can in your power to improve the situation.

So where to begin?

The best place to begin with diabetes is to go back to basics and follow your doctor's advice of eating healthy and exercising and also regularly monitoring your sugar levels. I would also recommend taking things a step further and taking a HB1Ac reading, so you can clearly see where your diabetes is at. This gives a baseline, as for a goal the goal is to try and improve your diabetes and get a HB1Ac on a regular basis as in maybe twice a year and keep on moving forward, always trying to get as close to the normal range as possible. If you get to the normal range than great and even if not, it's all good for the closer to the normal range the healthier you will be and the less likelihood of developing generative conditions.

On top of this take a look at the sections on super foods and herbs. Start taking all of the supplements listed on a daily basis, it just involves popping some pills which is easy to do. Many herb options will feel harder because they usual involve making an herbal tea and this can be a drag. So add one or two herbs, make it a habit and then add in some more. It takes 21 days to make a habit, so if you try too many things at once, chances are that you will drop out after a week or two. A very good place to start is in making yourself a mug of ginger tea a day as it is a great restorative. When a person has diabetes their body has become weekend energetically and it is necessity to take a tonic to build it back up.

Ginger tea can really help to build up your body over time, so it is a good starting point!

Regarding the different exercises and pranayama's which have been outlined, I would recommend that you take one exercise and one pranayama and stat doing them every day. After 21 days add in another exercise and the second pranayama. Then after another 21 days add in another Hatha or Taoist yoga exercise. The idea been to add these exercises in so slowly, that you don't find any difficulty. Simply add in one or two good exercises or habits every three weeks and over a period of months great things can occur!

Regarding acupressure, make a point of trying out some acupressure from day one and doing it for fifteen minutes a day as acupressure will really help.

So to summarise:

- **From day One** – Watch your diet and start exercising. Start acupressure for fifteen minutes every day. Start one pranayama and one Hatha or Taoist yoga exercise. Start taking supplements and start with one or two herbs.

- **After 21 days** add in another Taoist yoga or hatha yoga exercise and another pranayama exercise. Add in another herb.

- **After another 21 days**, add in another herb and some more exercises.

- **Every month** try and add in something positive and helpful for your health.

Of course you don't have to follow this suggested plan, the idea in writing out such a plan is simply to get you thinking, for its very easy to read a book like this and try out everything for two or three days and then stop. So if we want to reverse diabetes, begin by realising that the core cause of diabetes is degeneration within your physical and energetic health. You can blame it on genetics and lifestyle, but ultimately speaking your body has become weaker and is now out of balance. So to rebalance your body, you have to think in the long term as to in how can you restore health? How can you bring back vigour? How can you rejuvenate?

So when we think in terms of rejuvenation, then we move away from attempting to reverse diabetes with cheap tricks, which we read on the internet somewhere and instead we start taking things seriously and realise that our body's are out of synch and that we have to spend months, possibly even years slowly rejuvenating our bodies and bringing them back into a balanced state. When we take this approach, it becomes possible to reverse just about any health condition, because we are healing ourselves!

But be warned this is not an easy or quick trick. Yes you can make a great improvement to your blood sugar levels, within a few weeks, but to reverse your diabetes will taking many months or even years for most people to slowly rebalance things and bring increased vigour back into their bodies. And from a

TCM perspective, diabetes represents a weakness sin the body, degeneration and a healing has to take place, so that the body can rejuvenate itself and return back to a normal state of health. To do this is patient. Also buy yourself a diary or start noting things down electronically. Record your present HB1Ac levels and your daily fasting blood sugars and then over time work towards a general improvement.

Finally this book is not the last word on reversing diabetes, rather the purpose of this book has been to give you some tools and also to get you thinking about your diabetes and how to improve it. There are many different strategies, super foods and herbs which will help you to reverse your diabetes, if you stick at it over a long period of time!

Most importantly start today and be both patient and persistent and you will see not just short-term improvement, but also over the medium and long-term, not only will your diabetic symptoms improve, but also your overall health and wellbeing will improve along with it!

Free Gift

Grab Free Books!!!!!!!!

As a way of saying thank you for downloading this book I would like to give you two free books, which are available exclusively for my readers. The free book "Juicing for Health – 35 Juicing Recipes for Everyday Health Problems", is packed full of useful healthy juice recipes and Success Hacks - 31 Mind-Set Hacks to Increase Productivity and Career Success, is packed full of helpful mind hacks for developing a more dynamic and enjoyable lifestyle!

Please go to http://www.healbodymindandspirit.com/sign-up-page/ and sign up to my subscriber list and you shall receive the free book links via email.